THE POWERBUILDING BLUEPRINT

12-Week Roadmap to Add Muscle Size and Shatter PRs

By Todd Henry

DISCLAIMER:

IT IS STRONGLY RECOMMENDED THAT YOU CONSULT WITH YOUR PHYSICIAN BEFORE BEGINNING ANY DIET OR EXERCISE PROGRAM. EVEN IF YOU HAVE NO KNOWN HEALTH PROBLEMS, IT IS ADVISABLE TO CONSULT YOUR PHYSICIAN(S) BEFORE MAKING MAJOR CHANGES TO YOUR LIFESTYLE. THE MATERIAL CONTAINED IN THIS DIET AND EXERCISE PROGRAM IS PROVIDED FOR EDUCATIONAL AND INFORMATIONAL PURPOSES ONLY AND IS NOT INTENDED AS MEDICAL ADVICE. THE INFORMATION CONTAINED IN THIS PROGRAM SHOULD NOT BE USED TO DIAGNOSE OR TREAT ANY ILLNESS. ALL INFORMATION IS INTENDED FOR YOUR GENERAL KNOWLEDGE ONLY AND IS NOT A SUBSTITUTE FOR MEDICAL ADVICE OR TREATMENT FOR SPECIFIC MEDICAL CONDITIONS. THE INFORMATION IN THIS PROGRAM HAS NOT BEEN EVALUATED BY THE FDA AND IS NOT INTENDED TO DIAGNOSE, TREAT, CURE OR PREVENT ANY DISEASE, METABOLIC DISORDER OR HEALTH PROBLEMS. YOU SHOULD SEEK PROMPT MEDICAL CARE FOR ANY SPECIFIC HEALTH ISSUES.

AUTHOR'S DISCLAIMER:

THE AUTHOR IS NOT A DOCTOR. THE ADVICE PROVIDED HEREIN IS BASED ON YEARS OF PRACTICAL APPLICATION, BOTH WITH RESPECT TO THE AUTHOR'S OWN HEALTH AND PHYSIQUE, AS WELL AS THOSE OF OTHERS. ANY RECOMMENDATION THE AUTHOR MAKES TO YOU REGARDING DIET AND EXERCISE, INCLUDING SUPPLEMENTS AND HERBAL OR NUTRITIONAL TREATMENTS MUST BE DISCUSSED BETWEEN YOU AND YOUR PHYSICIAN(S)

Table of Contents

Introduction

Strength training has become a divided activity. Bodybuilding, powerlifting, cross fit, Olympic weightlifting, you name it. Where there is a category, there are respective silos with entire communities, industries and rules institutionalizing them.

Somewhere along the way, specific goals and agendas diluted the overall benefits of simple, effective weight training and the end result is an array of imbalanced lifters. Bodybuilders with superhuman physiques who can't squat 2x their body weight, powerlifters who can squat 4x their body weight but can't tie their shoes, cross fitters with "functional" strength but the maximal strength of a retired marathon runner, and so on.

The Powerbuilding Blueprint takes a step back from this nonsense and outlines a training method, a blueprint, for using basic, multi-joint movements to build maximal strength, and various assistance and accessory (isolation) lifts to stimulate hypertrophy, together. More basically, it combines the most effective training strategies for powerlifting and bodybuilding (an approach sometimes referred to as "powerbuilding"), in each workout, to maximize muscle size and strength gains from your time spent in the gym. It also produces incredibly well-rounded strength athletes.

The goal of this training program is simple: to give you a prescription for the best of both worlds - powerlifter strength and a bodybuilder's muscled, beach-ready physique.

Let me also say that this training comes with a precautionary warning: be prepared to train with intensity. Although the workouts are designed to be short (yet maximally effective), I won't sugar-coat this: you're going to be training *hard*. These are max-effort workouts.

With that in mind, please understand that nothing exceptional is built without extraordinary effort. If isolation work in front of the mirror at the pink and yellow gyms is all you're willing to commit, then I'm afraid this program isn't for you. In that case, there is no shame, just kindly forward this book to someone who's willing to go a bit further to achieve a lot more.

If you're still with me…congratulations. Let's get started!

PBB Philosophy

Before fad training programs and an exercise culture fixated on the secrets to 7-minute results and the like, traditional weight training consisted mostly of basic multi-joint movements with barbells and dumbbells. Workouts were hard work, weights were heavy and strength was as much an objective as a sculpted physique.

Since then, it certainly appears that things have changed, culturally. Gyms are often stocked with muscular bodybuilders (typically only from the waist up) who can't squat 2X their body weight. Form over function clearly dominates the landscape, unless you're a powerlifter, a rare champion of strength in a sport still mostly underground.

If you have had a propensity to prioritize muscle acquisition to the exclusion of performance, make no mistake -- strength is the essence of resistance training, and any training program that doesn't focus on building it is missing the mark. Even aesthetic bodybuilders ought to prioritize getting stronger, for a physique built of muscle with no utility is like a Lamborghini with a Volkswagen engine - should anyone care? Sure, it looks cool, but what can it do? Can it deliver the same thrill and exhilaration of a 600 horsepower V12?

The PBB training system will build both a muscular physique and impressive strength, just like old school bodybuilders and modern-day powerlifters who combine(d) impressive size and strength, using the same training principles.

Different Methods, Different Outcomes

In the same way that you can be big without being strong (which reminds me of a quote from Louie Simmons: "Big ain't strong. Strong is strong."), you can also be very strong without being equally big.

The reason for that boils down, basically, to the way that your body responds to different training stimuli. Powerlifters, due to their use of heavy loads (high percentages of their 1-repetition maxes or "1RMs") at low volume (sets/reps), get very strong through neurological changes and the type of hypertrophy (growth) they experience, which tends to be myofibrillar. Myofibrillar hypertrophy is an increase in the size and density of contractile muscle tissue (myofibrils), which adds to muscular strength.

Bodybuilders, by contrast, typically train with significantly lower percentages of their 1RMs at higher volumes, a training style that produces a greater degree of sarcoplasmic (and overall) hypertrophy. Sarcoplasmic hypertrophy reflects an increase in non-contractile muscle cell volume via an elevation in sarcoplasmic fluid, without an associated gain in muscular strength.[1] It is for this reason that bodybuilders are often not nearly as strong, pound-for-pound, as powerlifters, Olympic weightlifters or strongman competitors, despite, in some cases, superhuman appearances.

Optimally, then, a hybrid training approach targeting muscle size and strength by taking advantage of both powerlifting and bodybuilding training styles is ideal. This is what the PBB

training system does. It combines heavy loads with lower volume
at the beginning of each workout with moderate weights at higher
volume later in the workout, providing ideal training stimuli
for both muscle and strength gains.

Let's get to the details.

PBB Training

The program uses a 3-day/week schedule, beginning on Monday and
concluding on Friday (i.e. M-W-F), and is designed to be
performed in 12-16 week cycles (12 weeks represents the standard
template, but if you're peaking for an event such as a
powerlifting meet, there is an optional 4-week preparatory
block).

Additionally, every fourth week of the program is a "deload"
week. The primary goal of periodic deloading is to temporarily
back off heavy weights for the purpose of giving your central
nervous system (CNS), as well as your body – muscles and joints
– a rest, and priming them for future work. This feature of the
program is one I believe to be essential for staying healthy
week-after-week and cycle-after-cycle, particularly for older
lifters whose recuperative abilities are a fraction of what they
once were.

(The ideology behind "deloading" is best represented by Dr.
Vladimir Zatsiorsky's "Two-Factor Theory," which posits that
potential sport performance varies periodically based on the
balance between an athlete's "fitness gain" and "fatigue"
arising from his or her workouts. Through scheduled deloads,
cumulative fatigue is reduced and athletic performance is
increased.[2] Also, of particular interest to bodybuilders, studies
have shown that short-term deloads can lead to increases in both
growth hormone and testosterone, thus priming your body for
anabolic processes after normal training resumes.[3])

Each workout is broken down into a main lift, represented by the letter "**A**", an assistance lift ("**B**") and an accessory/finisher ("**C**"), performed in alphabetical order (A, B, C).

The overall set/rep scheme for the 12-16 weeks is structured as follows:

<u>Weeks 1-4</u>

A (Main lift) – 2 (work) sets x 4 reps

B (Assistance) – 5 sets x 10 reps

C (Accessory) – 3 sets x 12 reps

<u>Weeks 5-8</u>

A – 2 sets x 3 reps

B – 5 sets x 10 reps

C – 3 sets x 11 reps

<u>Weeks 9-12</u>

A – 2 sets x 2 reps

B – 5 sets x 10 reps

C – 3 sets x 10 reps

<u>Weeks 13-16 (Optional)</u>

A – 2 sets x 1 reps

B – 5 sets x 10 reps

C – 3 sets x 9 reps

Main Lifts ("A")

The main lifts will build tremendous strength, and consist of the squat, bench press and deadlift. They are performed on the following days:

Monday – Deadlift

Wednesday – Bench press

Friday – Squat

These "Big 3" lifts weren't chosen at random. Aside from the standing overhead press (which is an assistance lift on bench day, as you'll see below), they reflect the most effective lifts for muscle and strength acquisition. Every strength athlete, not just powerlifters, should be making the squat, bench and deadlift the centerpiece of their programs. And so it is with PBB.

As you dive into the program, you'll notice that the "A" lifts get heavier at lower volume (fewer reps) over the 12-16 week cycle. In general, weights each week are calculated as a percentage of your *projected* 1RM for each main lift at the end of the 12 or 16 weeks, not your current 1RM. However, the first time you train with this program, I strongly encourage you to use your current 1RM to determine your training weights, since I believe that a conservative approach to beginning a new program is a solid principle to follow. (In other words, start *slowly*.)

After each cycle (12 or 16 weeks), test your new 1RMs and then add reasonable increments to them in order to project your future 1RMs after the cycle you're planning, and use these projected maxes to determine your weights for the upcoming cycle.

For example, let's say your current squat max is 405. You'll plan your squat weights for your first cycle based on 405 (so, week 1 work sets will be performed with 275 - 405 x 67.5%, rounded to the nearest 5 pounds, and so on throughout the 12 or 16 weeks in accordance with the percentages outlined in the program). Then, after the cycle, you test your strength, and let's say that your new max is 425.

For the next cycle, your goal is to add another 20 pounds to your squat, so you set your projected max at 445, and base your weights on it. When you test your strength at the end of that cycle, you'll shoot for 100% of 445, which of course is a 445-lb. squat attempt.

See "Planning Training Cycles" below for more detail on periodization.

Assistance Lifts ("B")

Assistance lifts are intended to build the main lifts by training the muscles and (occasionally) movement patterns involved in the main lift. In the PBB program, they also serve to stimulate hypertrophy.

Weights for the "B" movements are not progressive by design in the program, since they're intended to build the main lifts and induce hypertrophy, not maximize strength. Hence the label "assistance." (The same goes for the "C" exercises.)

There is great variety with respect to assistance lift selection. For purposes of introducing you to this program, I've selected the assistance lift to perform for each workout over the first 12-16 weeks, but please understand that you can substitute these for myriad others.

For simplicity, I recommend following the program as outlined below, but for subsequent cycles (I'll discuss more thoroughly, below, how to plan training cycles), feel free to perform the following assistance lifts for variety and to address specific weaknesses (as they become clear):

Squat/Deadlift Assistance Exercises

Glute Ham Raises (GHR): GHRs are excellent for building posterior chain (lower back, glutes and hamstrings) size and strength. Many gyms don't have GHR equipment, which is unfortunate, as they truly are one of the most effective lifts for building the squat and deadlift. If you have access to a GHR, I strongly recommend including them into your assistance work.

Leg Press: Popular in many gyms (mostly because it's easier than squatting), the leg press is a good exercise for developing quad size and strength. Make sure you use a full range of motion and avoid using too much weight. No matter how much you load the leg press, it's never impressive.

Reverse Hyperextensions: The reverse hyper ranks alongside the GHR for building your posterior chain. Additionally, it's a great way to decompress the spine and, as such, is often used as a rehabilitation (or "prehab"/injury prevention) exercise. Elongating the spinal column relieves pressure on spinal discs, and enables spinal fluid to bathe the discs with oxygen and nutrients to speed recovery.

Good mornings: Perform these with a variety of bars, including:

- Safety squat bar

- Buffalo bar

- Cambered bar

- Straight bar

The good morning, performed correctly (find a reputable YouTube video), is one of the best exercises to build the low back, glutes and hamstrings, with tremendous carryover to the squat and deadlift.

Bent-over Rows: Great for developing the upper back and deadlift lockout strength. Also, there's no special equipment requirement with this lift. Load a barbell and get rowing. (Oh – and ditch the straps… Build grip strength/forearm size instead.)

Safety Squat Bar Squat: Specialty bars can not only add great variety to your lifting, but are also typically designed for assistance work. Squatting with a SSB is a humbling experience, as it really loads the low back, glutes and hamstrings (the primary squatting muscles).

Cambered Bar Squat: As with the SSB squat, the cambered bar squat is performed with a specialty (cambered) bar, and the altered placement of your hands, combined with the lower position of the weight, creates a great challenge for the musculature of

the low back. Stability can also be difficult with the cambered bar, building strength in the stabilizers.

Bench Press Assistance Exercises

Standing Overhead Press: More than any other exercise, this lift has added the most to my bench press, and it will carryover for you as well. Some would argue (myself included) that the standing press is a better measure of upper body strength than the bench, and anyone who's trained it would be hard pressed to disagree. This lift could easily replace the bench as the main lift, but we'll stay true to convention and use it as an assistance lift to build the bench instead. The press will train your shoulders, back, core and lower body.

Dumbbell Standing Overhead Press: Trains the same muscles and movement patterns as the barbell overhead press, but also imparts a level of instability in the movement, and provides an additional degree of freedom with the weight path. Experiment with different grips and dumbbell paths.

Dumbbell Bench Press: Performed at any angle (incline, flat, decline), these are excellent for developing the stabilizer muscles of the shoulder (given the instability of dumbbells vs. a barbell), and as with the dumbbell overhead press, enables additional leeway for various grips and movement patterns.

Board Press: Benching off 1-, 2-, 3- or 4-boards are intended to build lockout power in the bench, and are great for triceps strength and hypertrophy. Some say that these are only beneficial only for geared/equipped lifters, but I disagree. Anyone can benefit from bigger, stronger triceps.

Swiss Bar Bench: The Swiss bar is a specialty bar for the bench press that is designed with neutral grips at varying widths. I use this bar regularly to build my bench while alleviating much of the stress on my shoulders (it can be used as a rehab bar for that purpose as well). The neutral grip is great for triceps size and strength development.

Dips: Dips train the triceps, shoulders and chest, and build remarkable pressing power. Do these weighted or simply with body weight – they're effective either way.

Accessory Exercises ("C")

Accessory lifts in the PBB program are intended for hypertrophy training, and as such, are performed in the higher rep range (9-12). They're mostly isolation exercises typically used by bodybuilders because, as the name implies, they're quite effective at targeting specific muscles for growth.

While a more fleshed-out listing of accessory work might be akin to smashing a walnut with a sledgehammer (these are the lifts that pervade the weight rooms of commercial gyms everywhere and I'm sure you're aware of them), I'll bullet a few below:

Curls: Performed with either a barbell or dumbbell, they train the biceps. Variations included hammer curls (great for strengthening the distal biceps tendon, which is important for alternate-grip deadlifting), concentration curls, spider curls, etc.

Triceps Pushdown: These isolate and work the triceps.

Triceps Extension/Skull Crushers: Also train the triceps. Do a few high-rep sets of these, and you'll be feeling it for days.

Leg Curls: Leg curls train the hamstrings, and can actually be used as an assistance lift because they're quite effective. I've categorized here as an accessory movement because it's an isolation lift.

Leg Extension: As with the leg curl, this is a quadriceps isolation exercise effective for hypertrophy, but potentially hard on the knees. Use your judgment to determine if the cost/benefit computes favorably.

Planning Training Cycles

As noted above, your first 12- or 16-week cycle should be based on your current 1RMs. For the purpose of illustration, let's continue to use 405 for your current squat max. Your first squat cycle would look like the table on the following page. (Of course, this same methodology applies for the bench press and deadlift as well. For illustrative purposes, we're just looking at a hypothetical squat cycle.)

WEEK	EXERCISE	SETS	REPS	WEIGHT (LBS)
1	SQUAT	2	4	275
2	SQUAT	2	4	285
3	SQUAT	2	4	295
4	SQUAT (DELOAD)	2	4	225
5	SQUAT	2	3	295, 305
6	SQUAT	2	3	305, 315
7	SQUAT	2	3	315, 325
8	SQUAT (DELOAD)	2	3	225, 235
9	SQUAT	2	2	325, 335
10	SQUAT	2	2	335, 355
11	SQUAT	2	2	345, 355
12	SQUAT (DELOAD)	2	2	235, 245
13 (OPTIONAL)	SQUAT	1	1	355, 365
14 (OPTIONAL)	SQUAT	1	1	365, 375
15 (OPTIONAL)	SQUAT	1	1	375, 385
16 (OPTIONAL)	SQUAT (DELOAD)	1	1	245, 255
17	STRENGTH TEST	1	1	405+

Note, in the above example, a couple things:

If the optional weeks (13-16) were excluded, then the test week would be on week 13, rather than on week 17 as shown; and

"405+" is given as illustration to indicate that you'll test your strength by working up to a 1RM, which will constitute 100%+ of your existing PR (personal record).

Now, let's assume that you tested your strength, and hit a PR of 425. This new PR will become the basis for your projected max that will determine your training weights for the next cycle.

A reasonable projection for your PR after the following 12-16 weeks would be 445 (425 current PR plus a 20-pound improvement), which becomes your target squat at week 13 or 17 for the new cycle, which will look as follows:

WEEK	EXERCISE	SETS	REPS	WEIGHT (LBS)
1	SQUAT	2	4	300
2	SQUAT	2	4	310
3	SQUAT	2	4	325
4	SQUAT (DELOAD)	2	4	245
5	SQUAT	2	3	325, 335
6	SQUAT	2	3	335, 345
7	SQUAT	2	3	345, 355
8	SQUAT (DELOAD)	2	3	245, 255
9	SQUAT	2	2	355, 365
10	SQUAT	2	2	365, 380
11	SQUAT	2	2	380, 390
12	SQUAT (DELOAD)	2	2	255, 265
13 (OPTIONAL)	SQUAT	1	1	390, 400
14 (OPTIONAL)	SQUAT	1	1	400, 410
15 (OPTIONAL)	SQUAT	1	1	410, 425
16 (OPTIONAL)	SQUAT (DELOAD)	1	1	265, 280
17	STRENGTH TEST	1	1	445+

Peaking

Weeks 13-16, which are optional, are designed to prepare you for a strength competition, such as a powerlifting meet. If you've no interest in powerlifting or are training in the off-season, then simply skip these weeks and prepare for your next 12-week cycle, or, as I'll often do when a meet isn't marked on the calendar, you can go ahead with this peak and simply test your gym maxes during week 17 as if competing. I like to do this in order to stay sharp for when a meet pops up with little time to prepare.

During this phase, the objective of your workouts shifts from building strength and muscle to preparing you for *displaying* the strength you've gained throughout the training cycle.

This is an important distinction, and bears some reflection. Displaying maximum strength is a function of more than being strong. Being ready on meet day to demonstrate maximum strength through 1RMs requires a level of central nervous system preparedness that performing at or below 90% of your 1RM during your training cycle won't necessarily condition you for.

In order to perform maximally on meet day, you must prime your CNS to activate optimally, and your muscles and joints must be up for the task as well.

Thus, the peaking phase is designed to:

- Reduce fatigue (allow muscles and joints to recuperate from training cycle)

    ▢ Reinforce technique on the Big 3 (particularly at high % of 1RM)

    ▢ Practice 1RMs via progressively heavy singles

There are a couple things to note as you review the protocol for these weeks below:

In order to reduce fatigue, assistance and accessory volumes are scaled back, and accessory work is eliminated in week 16, which is a deload.

It is relatively conventional to deload the week prior to a meet (which this program prescribes at week 16), also for the purpose of allowing beat up muscles and joints to recover, really focus on technique, and prime the CNS for maximum performance on meet day.

WORKOUT 1

TYPE	EXERCISE	SETS	REPS	% 1RM
A	DEADLIFT	2	4	67.5
B	BENT OVER ROWS	5	10	
C	BARBELL CURLS	3	12	

WORKOUT 2

TYPE	EXERCISE	SETS	REPS	% 1RM
A	BENCH PRESS	2	4	67.5
B	OVERHEAD PRESS	5	10	
C	SKULL CRUSHERS	3	12	

WORKOUT 3

TYPE	EXERCISE	SETS	REPS	% 1RM
A	SQUAT	2	4	67.5
B	LEG PRESS	5	10	
C	LEG CURLS	3	12	

WORKOUT 1

TYPE	EXERCISE	SETS	REPS	% 1RM
A	DEADLIFT	2	4	70.0
B	BENT OVER ROWS	5	10	
C	BARBELL CURLS	3	12	

WORKOUT 2

TYPE	EXERCISE	SETS	REPS	% 1RM
A	BENCH PRESS	2	4	70.0
B	OVERHEAD PRESS	5	10	
C	SKULL CRUSHERS	3	12	

WORKOUT 3

TYPE	EXERCISE	SETS	REPS	% 1RM
A	SQUAT	2	4	70.0
B	LEG PRESS	5	10	
C	LEG CURLS	3	12	

WEEK 3

WORKOUT 1

TYPE	EXERCISE	SETS	REPS	% 1RM
A	DEADLIFT	2	4	72.5
B	BENT OVER ROWS	5	10	
C	BARBELL CURLS	3	12	

WORKOUT 2

TYPE	EXERCISE	SETS	REPS	% 1RM
A	BENCH PRESS	2	4	72.5
B	OVERHEAD PRESS	5	10	
C	SKULL CRUSHERS	3	12	

WORKOUT 3

TYPE	EXERCISE	SETS	REPS	% 1RM
A	SQUAT	2	4	72.5
B	LEG PRESS	5	10	
C	LEG CURLS	3	12	

WEEK 4 - DELOAD

WORKOUT 1

TYPE	EXERCISE	SETS	REPS	% 1RM
A	DEADLIFT	2	4	55.0
B	BENT OVER ROWS	5	10	
C	BARBELL CURLS	3	12	

WORKOUT 2

TYPE	EXERCISE	SETS	REPS	% 1RM
A	BENCH PRESS	2	4	55.0
B	OVERHEAD PRESS	5	10	
C	SKULL CRUSHERS	3	12	

WORKOUT 3

TYPE	EXERCISE	SETS	REPS	% 1RM
A	SQUAT	2	4	55.0
B	LEG PRESS	5	10	
C	LEG CURLS	3	12	

WEEK 5

WORKOUT 1

TYPE	EXERCISE	SETS	REPS	% 1RM
A	DEADLIFT	2	3	72.5, 75.0
B	BENT OVER ROWS	5	10	
C	BARBELL CURLS	3	11	

WORKOUT 2

TYPE	EXERCISE	SETS	REPS	% 1RM
A	BENCH PRESS	2	3	72.5, 75.0
B	OVERHEAD PRESS	5	10	
C	SKULL CRUSHERS	3	11	

WORKOUT 3

TYPE	EXERCISE	SETS	REPS	% 1RM
A	SQUAT	2	3	72.5, 75.0
B	LEG PRESS	5	10	
C	LEG CURLS	3	11	

WORKOUT 1

TYPE	EXERCISE	SETS	REPS	% 1RM
A	DEADLIFT	2	3	75.0, 77.5
B	BENT OVER ROWS	5	10	
C	BARBELL CURLS	3	11	

WORKOUT 2

TYPE	EXERCISE	SETS	REPS	% 1RM
A	BENCH PRESS	2	3	75.0, 77.5
B	OVERHEAD PRESS	5	10	
C	SKULL CRUSHERS	3	11	

WORKOUT 3

TYPE	EXERCISE	SETS	REPS	% 1RM
A	SQUAT	2	3	75.0, 77.5
B	LEG PRESS	5	10	
C	LEG CURLS	3	11	

WORKOUT 1

TYPE	EXERCISE	SETS	REPS	% 1RM
A	DEADLIFT	2	3	77.5, 80.0
B	BENT OVER ROWS	5	10	
C	BARBELL CURLS	3	11	

WORKOUT 2

TYPE	EXERCISE	SETS	REPS	% 1RM
A	BENCH PRESS	2	3	77.5, 80.0
B	OVERHEAD PRESS	5	10	
C	SKULL CRUSHERS	3	11	

WORKOUT 3

TYPE	EXERCISE	SETS	REPS	% 1RM
A	SQUAT	2	3	77.5, 80.0
B	LEG PRESS	5	10	
C	LEG CURLS	3	11	

WEEK 8 - DELOAD

WORKOUT 1

TYPE	EXERCISE	SETS	REPS	% 1RM
A	DEADLIFT	2	3	55.0, 57.5
B	BENT OVER ROWS	5	10	
C	BARBELL CURLS	3	11	

WORKOUT 2

TYPE	EXERCISE	SETS	REPS	% 1RM
A	BENCH PRESS	2	3	55.0, 57.5
B	OVERHEAD PRESS	5	10	
C	SKULL CRUSHERS	3	11	

WORKOUT 3

TYPE	EXERCISE	SETS	REPS	% 1RM
A	SQUAT	2	3	55.0, 57.5
B	LEG PRESS	5	10	
C	LEG CURLS	3	11	

WORKOUT 1

TYPE	EXERCISE	SETS	REPS	% 1RM
A	DEADLIFT	2	2	80.0, 82.5
B	BENT OVER ROWS	5	10	
C	BARBELL CURLS	3	10	

WORKOUT 2

TYPE	EXERCISE	SETS	REPS	% 1RM
A	BENCH PRESS	2	2	80.0, 82.5
B	OVERHEAD PRESS	5	10	
C	SKULL CRUSHERS	3	10	

WORKOUT 3

TYPE	EXERCISE	SETS	REPS	% 1RM
A	SQUAT	2	2	80.0, 82.5
B	LEG PRESS	5	10	
C	LEG CURLS	3	10	

WEEK 10

WORKOUT 1

TYPE	EXERCISE	SETS	REPS	% 1RM
A	DEADLIFT	2	2	82.5, 85.0
B	BENT OVER ROWS	5	10	
C	BARBELL CURLS	3	10	

WORKOUT 2

TYPE	EXERCISE	SETS	REPS	% 1RM
A	BENCH PRESS	2	2	82.5, 85.0
B	OVERHEAD PRESS	5	10	
C	SKULL CRUSHERS	3	10	

WORKOUT 3

TYPE	EXERCISE	SETS	REPS	% 1RM
A	SQUAT	2	2	82.5, 85.0
B	LEG PRESS	5	10	
C	LEG CURLS	3	10	

WORKOUT 1

TYPE	EXERCISE	SETS	REPS	% 1RM
A	DEADLIFT	2	2	85.0, 87.5
B	BENT OVER ROWS	5	10	
C	BARBELL CURLS	3	10	

WORKOUT 2

TYPE	EXERCISE	SETS	REPS	% 1RM
A	BENCH PRESS	2	2	85.0, 87.5
B	OVERHEAD PRESS	5	10	
C	SKULL CRUSHERS	3	10	

WORKOUT 3

TYPE	EXERCISE	SETS	REPS	% 1RM
A	SQUAT	2	2	85.0, 87.5
B	LEG PRESS	5	10	
C	LEG CURLS	3	10	

WEEK 12 - DELOAD

WORKOUT 1

TYPE	EXERCISE	SETS	REPS	% 1RM
A	DEADLIFT	2	2	57.5, 60.0
B	BENT OVER ROWS	5	10	
C	BARBELL CURLS	3	10	

WORKOUT 2

TYPE	EXERCISE	SETS	REPS	% 1RM
A	BENCH PRESS	2	2	57.5, 60.0
B	OVERHEAD PRESS	5	10	
C	SKULL CRUSHERS	3	10	

WORKOUT 3

TYPE	EXERCISE	SETS	REPS	% 1RM
A	SQUAT	2	2	57.5, 60.0
B	LEG PRESS	5	10	
C	LEG CURLS	3	10	

WEEK 13 [OPTIONAL] - PEAKING

WORKOUT 1

TYPE	EXERCISE	SETS	REPS	% 1RM
A	DEADLIFT	2	1	87.5, 90.0
B	BENT OVER ROWS	3	10	
C	BARBELL CURLS	2	9	

WORKOUT 2

TYPE	EXERCISE	SETS	REPS	% 1RM
A	BENCH PRESS	2	1	87.5, 90.0
B	OVERHEAD PRESS	3	10	
C	SKULL CRUSHERS	2	9	

WORKOUT 3

TYPE	EXERCISE	SETS	REPS	% 1RM
A	SQUAT	2	1	87.5, 90.0
B	LEG PRESS	3	10	
C	LEG CURLS	2	9	

WEEK 14 [OPTIONAL] - PEAKING

WORKOUT 1

TYPE	EXERCISE	SETS	REPS	% 1RM
A	DEADLIFT	2	1	90.0, 92.5
B	BENT OVER ROWS	3	10	
C	BARBELL CURLS	2	9	

WORKOUT 2

TYPE	EXERCISE	SETS	REPS	% 1RM
A	BENCH PRESS	2	1	90.0, 92.5
B	OVERHEAD PRESS	3	10	
C	SKULL CRUSHERS	2	9	

WORKOUT 3

TYPE	EXERCISE	SETS	REPS	% 1RM
A	SQUAT	2	1	90.0, 92.5
B	LEG PRESS	3	10	
C	LEG CURLS	2	9	

WEEK 15 [OPTIONAL] - PEAKING

WORKOUT 1

TYPE	EXERCISE	SETS	REPS	% 1RM
A	DEADLIFT	2	1	92.5, 95.0
B	BENT OVER ROWS	3	10	
C	BARBELL CURLS	2	9	

WORKOUT 2

TYPE	EXERCISE	SETS	REPS	% 1RM
A	BENCH PRESS	2	1	92.5, 95.0
B	OVERHEAD PRESS	3	10	
C	SKULL CRUSHERS	2	9	

WORKOUT 3

TYPE	EXERCISE	SETS	REPS	% 1RM
A	SQUAT	2	1	92.5, 95.0
B	LEG PRESS	3	10	
C	LEG CURLS	2	9	

WEEK 16 [OPTIONAL] – PEAKING [DELOAD]

WORKOUT 1

TYPE	EXERCISE	SETS	REPS	% 1RM
A	DEADLIFT	2	1	60.0, 62.5
B	BENT OVER ROWS	3	10	

WORKOUT 2

TYPE	EXERCISE	SETS	REPS	% 1RM
A	BENCH PRESS	2	1	60.0, 62.5
B	OVERHEAD PRESS	3	10	

WORKOUT 3

TYPE	EXERCISE	SETS	REPS	% 1RM
A	SQUAT	2	1	60.0, 62.5
B	LEG PRESS	3	10	

WEEK 17 - TEST STRENGTH [MAX ATTEMPT]

TEST DAY 1

TYPE	EXERCISE	SETS	REPS	% 1RM
A	DEADLIFT	1	1	100.0+

TEST DAY 2

TYPE	EXERCISE	SETS	REPS	% 1RM
A	BENCH PRESS	1	1	100.0+

TEST DAY 3

TYPE	EXERCISE	SETS	REPS	% 1RM
A	SQUAT	1	1	100.0+

Q: I DON'T SEE WARM-UPS ADDRESSED IN THE PROGRAM...HOW DO I PROPERLY WARM UP?

Warm-up sets essentially serve two purposes: (1) "loosen" soft and connective tissues to prepare them for activity, and (2) activate and prime your CNS for your work sets.

Of these, the second objective is the most important for performance, and the one managed most poorly by the average lifter.

After the first set or two, your warm-ups should be performed with low reps, descending as your warm-up weights increase. Let me illustrate a typical warm-up routine for a squat workout in which I'll train at roughly 90% of my 1RM:

Bar x 10
135 x 5
225 x 3
315 x 2
405 x 2
495 x 1
585 x 1
635 x 1

Work sets (@ ~90%):
655 x 2 x 2
675 x 2 x 2

You'll notice that I'll start out with just the bar and perform
10 reps. This is to get my muscles and joints warm and prepared
for activity. The subsequent warm-up sets are to progressively
activate and prime the CNS for maximal weights, jumping up in
weight by the addition of 45-lb plates. Notice that my rep
range is low (1-3), and my final two or three warm-up sets are
typically just singles. Any more work that this is simply
unnecessary and counterproductive.

Q: IS TRAINING 3 TIMES PER WEEK SUFFICIENT? I THOUGHT MORE OFTEN IS BETTER.

For the ideal balance of strength and hypertrophy, I've found 3-
4 workouts per week to be optimal. Training more frequently can
often limit strength gains because it doesn't allow sufficient
recovery from heavy lifting (especially with respect to the
nervous system, and as one ages, muscles and particularly
joints, which have a reduced capacity for recuperation).

During various periods of my own training, I've experimented
with 4 workouts per week, often during meet training cycles, and
this frequency generally ended up doing more harm than good when
weighing gains versus how beat up I'd be at the end of a
training cycle. Thus, a 3-day training schedule spread evenly
over the week has always seemed to work best for me, and I
believe it works very well for the majority of lifters,
especially those training without the use of performance-
enhancing drugs (PEDs).

WHAT IS THE CORRECT TEMPO TO APPLY TO THE LIFTS?

If you're unfamiliar with tempo, it refers to the amount of time (typically expressed in seconds) it takes to perform the three phases of a lift: (1) concentric, (2) isometric and (3) eccentric. The way this is often expressed is as follows (for example): 3-1-3.

In this example, you'd perform the lift at a pace of 3 seconds raising the weight, followed by a 1 second pause, and then 3 seconds to lower the weight.

In my view, any approach in which you're required to count the duration of repetitions is losing the forest for the trees. Generally speaking, time under tension is an important factor in hypertrophy, but I suggest using the number of repetitions as the driver. Based on researching suggesting a dose-response relationship between training volume and hypertrophy[4], it has generally been theorized that sets lasing 30-60 seconds in duration are most effective for muscle size increases.

So, rather than performing 10 repetitions at 3-6 seconds each (where each phase of the rep is counted), I recommend simply using a stopwatch (one time) to determine how many repetitions you perform in a 30-60 second interval (following the guideline below for rep speed). Then perform that many reps per set when you want to add variety to your hypertrophy training.

Now, what rep speed do I recommend? Well, I've found that if your strategy is to build muscle and strength (together) maximally, it's best to perform the concentric (raising) portion of a given lift as fast as possible (as weights increase, the bar speed will obviously drop markedly, but you'll still perform

the contraction at maximum *intended* speed), and lower the bar
under control.

Focus more on successfully completing each rep with respectable
form and "feeling" the weight (the mind/body connection is
important!), and less on how long you're raising and lowering
it.

Q: HOW LONG SHOULD I REST BETWEEN SETS? DO I NEED TO USE A TIMER?

This is another concern that is largely subjective, but
generally, you will need to rest somewhere in the range of 3-5
minutes between sets of your main ("A") lifts, 2-3 minutes
between sets of your assistance ("B") lifts, and as little as
60-90 seconds for your accessory work ("C" lifts).

As a rule, the compound, multi-joint exercises performed above
70% of your 1RM will require the most rest between sets, while
isolation work will fall at the other end of the spectrum,
particularly if not performed to failure. For the latter,
resting only 1 minute between sets is often sufficient.

In the end, it's up to you to determine when you're ready for
the next set, which is an intuitive decision based on your level
of perceived "preparedness" for the upcoming set. Except for
the purpose described above, I don't normally recommend using a
stopwatch or other timing device to monitor your rest periods.
Lift when you're ready to perform at or close to 100%.

Deloading in this context refers to a planned, periodic use of lighter weights and also, occasionally, less volume to rest the CNS, muscles and joints.

I believe deloading every several weeks serves a few critical purposes, the benefits of which I've certainly seen in my own training. They are:

- Recuperation: As mentioned, the primary intent is recuperative (i.e. reduce cumulative "fatigue"). Week after week of heavy lifting takes a physical toll on your body, something that becomes increasingly apparent with age. At the time of this writing, I'm 41, and let me tell you…I don't recover like I used to (I've been training in a goal-oriented way for over 25 years). The specter of substantial injury is always a looming factor in my programming.

- Central nervous system: This could also be labelled as recuperative, but instead of relating to the soft and connective tissues, this recovery is with respect to the master control center responsible for activating muscle: the central nervous system. For years, I inevitably found that whenever I'd take a short break from training (a week or less), I'd return to the gym feeling stronger than ever. I always chalked it up to the physical recovery of muscles and joints, but now realize the more significant reason for this apparent paradox was that the short break allowed

sufficient CNS recovery to prime activation upon my return.
This is an under-appreciated phenomenon in the training
world, and I ask you not to overlook it.

☐ Injury prevention: The logical extension of recovering
fully from training is the reduced likelihood of injury.
Over time, microscopic strains become small or minor
strains, which unattended become moderate strains, and so
on. Deloading allows the small stuff to heal before
becoming big stuff.

☐ Attitude: I'm rarely hungrier to lift with intensity than
after a week during which I've deliberately "held back"
(under 70% of 1RM). Lifting at high-intensity is a
prerequisite to my sanity, but if that's all I did, day in
and day out, I'm not sure I'd appreciate it as much or
glean the same level of therapeutic benefit from it.

☐ Technique: Deloading is a great time to work on perfecting
technique via muscle-memory. We all know that technique
erodes as the weights increase, so by practicing technique
with significant repetitions at lighter weights,
particularly on a periodic basis, you can help lock-in
correct movement patterns that will ultimately carry over
to heavier lifting. Remember that for proper technique,
weight training should be thought of as training movement
patterns, not individual muscles.

Note: Deload weeks aren't critical to this program (except for
the final deload week if you're peaking), which is designed to
work with or without them. However, it is my recommendation
that you observe them as outlined, for the above reasons.

Should you decide not to, simply skip each deload week and
continue with the weight progression as delineated.

Q: WHY ISN'T THERE A PROGRESSION FOR ASSISTANCE ("B") AND ACCESSORY ("C") LIFTS?

The meat and potatoes of this training program or any other for
building foundational muscle and strength are the core lifts:
squat, bench and deadlift. (The standing overhead press is in
this category as well, but I think of it more as a special
exercise for building the bench – and thus can be incorporated
into this program as a "B" lift.)

As such, there is a clear and effective progression involving
systematically heavier weights with descending repetitions for
the core lifts, leading up to the strength test following each
training cycle.

Assistance and accessory exercises, by their classification, are
not the central focus of the program. As noted above,
assistance exercises build the main lifts (and contribute to
hypertrophy), and accessory/isolation work is for hypertrophy.
Rather than program a progression for these lifts, select
weights that enable you to perform the prescribed number of
repetitions, while leaving a couple repetitions (1 or 2) in the
tank. Naturally, as you get stronger, these weights will
increase, but continue to live by the rule of selecting the
weight that enables you perform the reps with 1 or 2 in reserve.

I'll repeat: do not train these to momentary concentric failure.
You'll provide more than enough stimulus for growth by stopping
a rep or two short of failure.

Q: HOW DO I DETERMINE MY PROJECTED 1RM FOR THE NEXT TRAINING CYCLE?

With hesitation, I decided not to embed a rule into the program for determining your projected 1RMs for each training cycle.

The reason is because I believe it's very subjective, and ultimately a matter of your judgment after each and every 12- or 16-week training block. After you test your strength in either week 13 or 17, you'll have updated PRs. It's then up to you to decide your targets for the next strength test (at week 13 or 17 of the next training block), and base your weights for the upcoming cycle on those targets.

Personally, there have been 12-week cycles in which I've projected 50-LB. PRs, and others where I've only forecasted 15-25 pound increases over my current maxes. After you graduate to an intermediate or advanced lifter (if you're not already), you'll be so attuned to your body and training momentum that these decisions are relatively easy.

For beginners, if you're forcing me to create a rule, I suggest raising your targets 25-50 pounds over your current squat and deadlift maxes, and 15-30 pounds over your bench max.

Eating for maximum muscle size and strength is straightforward: eat robustly. Preferably at macronutrient ratios that are favorable for muscle growth (which I'll cover briefly a bit later).

However, the challenge lies not in how to eat for gaining weight indiscriminately, but rather in how to gain quality lean muscle without adding pounds of body fat. Let me give you an example, with numbers, to illustrate more precisely what I mean by this.

Let's say (for the sake of easy math) that you are currently weighing in at 200 lbs with 15% body fat. This means that your body consists of approximately 170 lbs of lean mass (200 x 85%) and 30 lbs of fat (200 x 15%).

Now let's say that in order to fuel maximum muscle gains, you go on an eating binge and, as a result of intense weight training and excess calories ("acute overfeeding"), you gain 8 lbs over the next 4 weeks.

According to (limited) scientific study, in what would probably constitute the *best case scenario*, that 8 lbs would be composed of around 70% fat-free mass and 30% fat, meaning that you will have added 5.6 lbs of lean mass and 2.4 lbs of fat to your body. Given that, your body comp will break down as follows:

- Lean mass: 175.6 lbs (up from 170 -- good)
- Fat mass: 32.4 lbs (up from 30 -- not good)
- Body fat %: 15.6% (up from 15.0% -- not good)

So, you have busted your ass for the last 4 weeks in the gym, and you have gorged on food, which is often only pleasant for the first few days, after which it becomes both uncomfortable and inconvenient (the food prep alone can be a killer).

Your reward is 5.6 lbs of new lean mass, but at a cost of an extra 2.4 lbs of fat, which unfortunately raised your body fat from 15.0% to 15.6%.

(Note: In this hypothetical scenario, the reason your body fat percentage increased is because you gained weight in a 70/30 ratio, which appears to be the best case scenario supported by scientific study[4]; therefore, if your starting body fat percentage is less than 30%, then this new weight will increase your body fat percentage, and vice versa if your starting body fat percentage is above 30%.)

See the problem?

The bottom line is, without a reduction in body fat percentage (or at least staying flat), that 5 lb gain in new muscle you worked so hard for is likely to go unnoticed, and not contribute to your goal of improving your physique.

Why? Well, because ultimately, it is the ratio of lean to fat mass (i.e. your body fat percentage) that determines how you look.

For muscle to be attractive, you have to see it unadulterated by layers of fat. Simply having more muscle than the average guy or gal typically doesn't contribute to your looking more

athletic and aesthetically pleasing, unless it's coupled with a
sufficiently low body fat percentage.

Otherwise, you'll just take up more space.

A Quick Word on Calorie-Counting

Now that you understand that the goal isn't simply to gain weight, but rather to gain lean muscle without gaining fat (and perhaps even to reduce it), let's talk about how to actually achieve it.

First, let me say that I don't buy the old calories-in vs. calories-out conventional wisdom as it relates to body composition. This is the model that says that in order to lose a pound of fat, you have to reduce your calorie intake (through diet) or increase calorie burning (through exercise) by 3,500 calories (relative to your calorie requirement), because 1 lb of fat contains 3,500 calories. The theory holds for gaining muscle as well (i.e. you need to create a calorie surplus of approximately 3,500 calories to build a lb of muscle).

Nonsense.

Many factors influence body composition and how nutrients are used and stored by your body, many of which are completely independent of the calorie content of food.

For example, anabolic steroids and other performance-enhancing drugs typically cause dramatic increases in lean muscle without adding a single calorie to your diet, because of the effect that they have on your physiology (and nutrient metabolism).

Prednisone, the very popular anti-inflammatory drug that physicians dispense for even the most benign conditions, has the opposite effect on body composition. It often contributes to

rapid and substantial gains in body fat, yet it contains zero
calories.[5]

What these drugs do, in part, is affect the way your body
partitions nutrients (that is, whether nutrients and calories
get directed to lean storage compartments like muscle cells, or
unsightly fat storage compartments).

In that way, they're not unique. Many nutrients found in common
foods have "drug like" actions as well, including nutrient
partitioning, which is why the old, straight calories-in vs.
calories-out mathematical model is largely nonsense. Food
quality (what you eat) is just as important as food quantity
(how much you eat).

So, why do I say that conventional wisdom is "largely," and not
"completely," nonsense?

Well, because calories are still an important component of any
physique improvement strategy, and as you'll see in a moment,
manipulating them slightly can work to our advantage. Without
the use of performance-enhancing drugs, or even certain
nutraceuticals, to preferentially shuttle nutrients toward lean
muscle building and away from body fat depots, you will
unfortunately need to manipulate calorie consumption through
diet to move the meter in the right direction.

The reason I wanted to "set the record straight" on the old
conventional wisdom is to put calorie-counting into perspective:
Do NOT obsess over it. The level of precision implied by
conventional wisdom is a fallacy that somehow never dies -- it's
the cockroach of nutritional science. The truth is, as long as

you're staying within reasonable margins of what I'm about to
outline, you will achieve your goals without precise calorie
control.

Calorie Cycling

Generally, to optimize muscle growth without the use of powerful repartitioning agents like anabolic steroids, you would need to consistently consume more calories than your body burns in order to satisfy the additional energy demand of the muscle-building process.

At this point, I don't have to point out the inherent flaw in that strategy, for we now know that constantly being in an "overfed" state will lead to ugly fat accumulation over time, as a portion of excess calories will invariably divert to your body's 30 billion fat cells. Your body is programmed to do this in accordance with its evolutionary mandate to store vital energy for a potential future famine.

Most bodybuilders account for this dilemma by enduring periodic cycles of "gaining" and "cutting." Thus, one might deliberately overfeed for 12 weeks to pack on muscle, and then roll into a calorie-restricted diet for 12 weeks in an attempt to remove the fat acquired during the gaining phase, while preserving as much of the new muscle growth as possible. Then the cycle repeats.

That strategy can work for lifters using nutrient-partitioning drugs like anabolic steroids, because such agents tilt the scale rather dramatically in favor of muscle. But unfortunately for those who opt out of drug use, I'm sorry to say that protracted cycles of gaining and cutting do not yield great results. In the end, many lifters find that at best, they're at "break even" after repetitive cycles, where any weight acquired during gaining (including new muscle growth) is lost during the

subsequent cutting phase. In worse cases, net fat accumulation
results over time as more fat is picked up during the gaining
phase than is lost during the subsequent diet, and your physique
is actually worse off after each cycle.

Fortunately, there's a better way.

Instead of long cycles of over- and under-feeding, alternating
every other day between maintenance calories (the quantity that
theoretically maintains your body weight without loss or gain)
and 125% of maintenance calories will supply your body with
extra calories on a fairly regular basis without doing so in
perpetuity (which is ultimately the signal that instructs the
body to "switch priorities" over to fat storage).

In fact, a number of scientific studies have shown that "acute,"
or short-term overfeeding (consuming more calories than you
burn), leads initially to (substantial) lean body mass gains,
even among sedentary people who do not train with weights! This
favorable condition only lasts for about two weeks, however,
after which the body appears to abruptly change objectives and
begins to preferentially store fat.[6,7]

Thus, very modestly overfeeding on an every-other-day schedule
is a kind of dietary sleight-of-hand that will optimize your
metabolism toward your goal of gaining attractive lean muscle
without sabotage from fat accumulation.

Note that this strategy won't produce significant fat loss, but
it will ensure that you're able to support new muscle gains when
combined with the PBB training method, *without gaining fat along
with lean muscle.*

(Note that you could, however, achieve the flip-side of this
objective -- losing fat while preserving muscle -- by
alternating between 100% of maintenance calories and 75%.)

So, using this approach, your week would look something like
this:

Day 1: 100% (of maintenance calories)
Day 2: 125%
Day 3: 100%
Day 4: 125%
Day 5: 100%
Day 6: 125%
Day 7: 100%

Get it? It's very simple and relatively easy to follow, which
I'll demonstrate with sample menus in a few moments.

But first, let me break the overall nutrition plan down for you
into steps.

Eating for Your Goals

So, you now know the goal and have a rough idea on the methodology that will get you there, which I'll restate: acquire quality muscle without gaining fat. Here are the steps to do that:

1. a. Men: Multiply your body weight by 15 (This is your "maintenance" calorie level)

   b. Women: Multiply your body weight by 12 (This is your "maintenance" calorie level)

2. a. Men: Multiply your body weight by 18.75 (This is 125% of maintenance)

   b. Women: Multiply your body weight by 15 (This is 125% of maintenance)

3. Determine daily macros

4. Determine meal macros

5. Model your meal plan after the sample I provide below (if you're so inclined)

1 – MAINTENANCE CALORIES

This is easy. Determine approximately how many calories your body needs each day (to maintain stable weight) by multiplying your body weight in pounds by 15 if you're a man, or 12 if you're a woman.

So, for a 200-lb male (keeping the math simple), this would be 3,000 (200 x 15 - 3,000) calories per day. This level is considered your baseline. The assumption is, if you consume substantially more than this every day, you'll gain weight, and vice versa.

2 - SURPLUS CALORIES

Same idea, but instead of using 15 and 12 as the multipliers for men and women, respectively, you're going to use 18.75 and 15, respectively. So for our hypothetical 200-lb male, this would be 3,750 calories (200 x 18.75).

3 - DAILY MACROS

A lot of people in the fitness world get hung up on "macros," or macronutrient ratios. This means the proportion of your total calories that come from each of the three macronutrients in the diet: protein, carbohydrates and fat.

I do believe that macronutrient ratios are important (and part of the food "quality" vs. "quantity" discussion above), but like calorie-counting, I don't believe you should get hung up on them.

The truth is, there is no magic ratio that supports muscle building or fat loss, and anyone who contends otherwise is wrong (and probably disingenuous). However, there are general guidelines that you can follow that work well for most lifters.

With that in mind, here's what I recommend:

First, let protein requirement drive everything else. A rule of thumb that you should use as a starting point is to consume 1 gram of protein per pound of body weight, per day. So, again, using our 200-lb individual (this is not gender-specific), that would be 200 grams of protein per day.

Given that 200 grams equates to 800 calories (at 4 calories per gram), it follows that protein should constitute about 30% of your total daily calories (800 / 3,000 = 27%, so we'll round up).

Then, set dietary fat at 25% of total daily calories (another rule of thumb), and the remainder is fulfilled by carbohydrates (in this case, 45%). Obviously, we would simply this to 30/45/25.

Thus, in this example, our 200-lb hypothetical male lifter's daily macros (at the "maintenance" level) breakdown as follows:

- Protein: 30% of total calories, which equates to 900 calories, or 225 grams
- Carbohydrates: 45% of total calories, 1,350 calories, 337 grams
- Fats: 25% of total calories, 750 calories, 83 grams

(Note that protein and carbs contain 4 calories per gram, while dietary fats contain 9 calories per gram.)

Remember that there's no magic to this, but is intended to give you reasonable parameters for developing your daily nutrition plan. If each macro is off even significantly at the end of a given day but you've otherwise eaten in a manner consistent with your goals (clean, nutrient-dense foods within portion guidelines, etc.), then celebrate a victory, not a loss.

4 – MEAL MACROS

Let's talk about how many times per day you should eat.

The conventional wisdom on this topic is six meals per day for strength and physique athletes. Whether or not this is truly optimal is debatable, but I nevertheless recommend it anyway. Here are the most compelling reasons why:

- Eating every few hours during the day staves off hunger and therefore regulates appetite, a key component of nutritional success.

- More frequent meals means splitting your daily nutrient and calorie demands into smaller portions, aiding digestive comfort and *possibly* nutrient absorption; while evidence suggests that larger meals can typically be digested just fine, there's no question that for many folks, smaller portions means less bloating and discomfort after meals.

- Consuming protein every few hours delivers a steady supply of amino acids (which all dietary proteins get disassembled into) to your body. Amino acids serve innumerable vital functions in the body and are the so-called "building blocks" of protein. Since skeletal muscle consists primarily of protein and water, amino acids are essential to building muscle (by supplying the necessary material and, in certain cases, even signaling the construction).

- While the effect of frequent meals on insulin sensitivity is also debatable, consuming moderate amounts of quality carbohydrate every few hours ensures that your blood

glucose levels remain relatively stable, and you can mostly
avoid otherwise typical oscillations in energy levels
throughout the day.

With meal frequency in mind, let's continue with our example
nutrition plan for our 200-lb hypcthetical male lifter. From
above, here's a recap of the daily macros we determined:

Protein: 225 grams

Carbohydrates : 337 grams

Dietary fat: 83 grams

Now let's spread those daily targets evenly over six meals,
which looks like this:

At 2,400 Calories Per Day ("Maintenance")

Protein: 225 grams / 6 meals = 37.5 grams per meal

Carbohydrates: 337 grams / 6 meals = 56 grams per meal

Dietary fat: 80 grams / 6 meals = 13.33 grams per meal

(Obviously, these are guidelines, and we can round and
approximate.)

Now that we have meal macros at the "maintenance" level, let's
convert them to what our 200-lb lifter will need at 25% above
maintenance:

At 3,750 Calories Per Day ("Surplus")

Protein: 37.5 grams x 125% = 47 grams per meal (rounded)

Carbohydrates: 56 grams x 125% = 70 grams per meal

Dietary fat: 13 grams x 125% = 16 grams grams per meal (rounded)

5 - PUTTING IT ALL TOGETHER: SAMPLE DAILY MENUS

Below, I have detailed my actual meal plan for two particular days, one for a 100% day, and another for a 125% day. These happen (not coincidentally) to fit with our hypothetical 200-lb male lifter because, you guessed it, that fits my profile.

I am approximately 5'8'', 200 lbs, typically around 8% body fat. Sometimes I get leaner, but rarely do I rise above that body fat level, even at 41 years old (as of the time of this writing).

These sample days from my nutrition journal reflect very typical ones for me, as I don't vary much from day to day, week to week or even year to year. I'm a creature of habit, and consistency is what enables me to follow a solid nutritional strategy without much effort, and for the long run. (My nutrition has been pretty consistent for the last 25 years!)

That is not so say that you can't mix things up, and actually I encourage you to do so, but once you find what works for you, it's not uncommon to discover that consistency offers advantages of convenience that trumps your desire for variety.

In any case, I can't say this enough:

You do NOT have to copy these sample daily menus. They're intended, instead, to illustrate how the numbers above can translate into actual food. But these are just two of an infinite number of food (and supplement) combinations that can

work within the above guidelines. Ultimately, find "clean"
foods that you enjoy, and build out your menu around them.
That's how you'll set yourself up for success in the long run.

Lastly -- notice that the numbers are not perfect on either day.

With respect to the 100% day, instead of hitting precisely 30%
protein, 45% carbs and 25% fats on total calorie intake of 3,000
calories as outlined above (for the "maintenance" day), on this
particular day, I hit 36% protein, 41% carbs and 22% fats with
total calories of 2,962 -- pretty damn close enough.

On the 125% day, I hit 37% protein, 38% carbs and 24% fats with
total calories of 3,725, relative to targets of 30% protein, 45%
carbs, 25% fats and 3,750 total calories. Again, *close enough*.

Remember that there is no magic formula, and counting calories
is mostly unnecessary. After doing this for a while, you'll
intuitively know which foods to eat, and how much, to achieve
your goals.

(For example, very little effort went into "designing" the
sample menus below, which I did on the fly on those particular
days and not in advance, yet I hit total calories and macros
within relatively tight margins. This is, again, because I've
been pretty consistent for so long that tweaks from day-to-day
don't have to be belabored.)

So, without further ado:

100% Maintenance Day:

TIME	FOOD/DIETARY SUPPLEMENT	QTY	CALS	P (g)	C (g)	F (g)
6:00 a.m.	**BREAKFAST**					
	Protein Shake (Mixed in water):					
	Synergy XP™ Vanilla Cream protein powder	**1.5 scoops**	**182**	**37**	**4**	**2**
	1 Banana	**1**	**112**	**1**	**27**	**0**
	Almond butter	1 Tbs	**114**	**3**	**3**	**10**
	Instant Oatmeal (low-sugar apple cinnamon flavor)	**1 packet**	**122**	**3**	**24**	**1.5**
	MEAL TOTALS		**530**	**44**	**58**	**13.5**
9:00 a.m.	**MID-MORNING**					
	Perfect Bar™ (peanut butter flavor)	1 bar	**334**	**17**	**26**	**18**
	Greek yogurt (low-sugar blueberry flavor)	2 servings	**160**	**24**	**16**	**0**
	MEAL TOTALS		**494**	**41**	**42**	**18**
12:00 p.m.	**LUNCH**					
	Tuna sandwich:					
	Tuna (packed in water)	**1 can**	**105**	**24**	**0**	**1**

Whole-grain bread	2 slices	177	5	37	1
Salad with dark greens and avocado	Unlimited	130	0	10	10
MEAL TOTALS		412	29	47	12

3:00 p.m.	**MID-AFTERNOON**					

Omelet:

Whole eggs	2	129	12	0	9
Egg whites	6	48	12	0	0
Instant oatmeal (low-sugar apple cinnamon flavor)	1 packet	122	3	24	1.5
Piece of fruit: typically apple or orange	1	100	0	25	0
MEAL TOTALS		423	33	49	10.5

6:00 p.m.	**WORKOUT**

7:00 p.m.	**POST-WORKOUT NUTRITION SHAKE**

Protein Shake (Mixed in 12-14 oz. of cold water):

Synergy XP™ Vanilla Cream protein powder	1.5 scoops	191	37	4	3
Dextrose powder	1/3 cup	200	0	50	0
Creatine monohydrate	5 grams	0	0	0	0
MEAL TOTALS		391	37	54	3

8:00 p.m.	**DINNER**

Beef sirloin steak (fat-trimmed)	6 ounces	310	46	0	14
Starch (potatoes, rice, quinoa, multigrain bread, pasta, etc)	1 portion*	172	3	40	0

			CALS	P (g)	C (g)	F (g)
	Dark green veggies	Unlimited	40	0	10	0
	MEAL TOTALS		**522**	**49**	**50**	**14**

TIME	FOOD/DIETARY SUPPLEMENT	QTY	CALS	P (g)	C (g)	F (g)
11:00 p.m.	**BEDTIME**					
	Protein Shake (Mixed in 12-14 oz. of cold water):					
	Synergy XP™ Vanilla Cream protein powder	**1.5 scoops**	191	37	4	3
	MEAL TOTALS		**191**	**37**	**4**	**3**

		CALS	P (g)	C (g)	F (g)
DAILY TOTALS		**2,962**	**270**	**304**	**74**
% OF CALORIES		**100%**	**36%**	**41%**	**22%**

125% Maintenance Day:

TIME	FOOD/DIETARY SUPPLEMENT	QTY	CALS	P (g)	C (g)	F (g)
6:00 a.m.	**BREAKFAST**					

Protein Shake (Mixed in water):

Synergy XP™ Rich Chocolate protein powder	2 scoops	243	50	4	3
1 Banana	1	112	1	27	0
Almond butter	1 Tbs	114	3	3	10
Instant Oatmeal (low-sugar apple cinnamon flavor)	**2 packets**	**243**	**6**	**48**	**3**
MEAL TOTALS		**712**	**60**	**82**	**16**

9:00 a.m. MID-MORNING

Perfect Bar™ (peanut butter flavor)	**1 bar**	**334**	**17**	**26**	**18**
Greek yogurt (low-sugar blueberry flavor)	**2 servings**	**160**	**24**	**16**	**0**
MEAL TOTALS		**494**	**41**	**42**	**18**

12:00 p.m. LUNCH

Tuna melt sandwich:

Tuna (packed in water)	1 can	105	24	0	1
Cheese (reduced fat)	2 slices	102	10	2	6
Whole-grain bread	2 slices	177	5	37	1
Salad with dark greens and avocado	**Unlimited**	**130**	**0**	**10**	**10**
MEAL TOTALS		**514**	**39**	**49**	**18**

3:00 p.m. MID-AFTERNOON

Omelet:

Whole eggs	3	193.5	18	0	13.5

Egg whites	6	72	18	0	0
Instant oatmeal (low-sugar apple cinnamon flavor)	1 packet	122	3	24	1.5
Piece of fruit: typically apple or orange	1	100	0	25	0
MEAL TOTALS		487	39	49	15

6:00 p.m. **WORKOUT**

7:00 p.m. **POST-WORKOUT NUTRITION SHAKE**

Protein Shake (Mixed in 12-14 oz. of cold water):

Synergy XP™ Vanilla Cream protein powder	2 scoops	243	50	4	3
Dextrose powder	1/2 cup	300	0	75	0
Creatine monohydrate	5 grams	0	0	0	0
MEAL TOTALS		543	50	79	3

8:00 p.m. **DINNER**

Beef sirloin steak (fat-trimmed)	8 ounces	406	61	0	18
Starch (potatoes, rice, quinoa, multigrain bread, pasta, etc)	1 portion*	172	3	40	0
Dark green veggies	Unlimited	40	0	10	0
MEAL TOTALS		618	64	50	18

11:00 p.m. **BEDTIME**

Protein Shake (Mixed in 12-14 oz. of cold water):

Synergy XP™ Vanilla Cream protein powder	1.5 scoops	243	50	4	3

Almond butter	1 Tbs	114	3	3	10
MEAL TOTALS		**357**	**53**	**7**	**13**

		P	C	F
DAILY TOTALS	**3,725**	**346**	**358**	**101**
% OF CALORIES	**100%**	**37%**	**38%**	**24%**

Legend:

   P = Protein

   C = Carbohydrates

   F = Fats

   g = grams

Optimizing 100 / 125 Anabolic Cycling

Before we move on, there are a couple key items on the Sample Daily Menus worth discussing, as their inclusion will produce optimal results.

NUTRITIONAL SUPPLEMENTS

You will notice that I use nutritional supplements, sometimes virtually as entire meals. I am aware that there is a community of "food purists" out there who believe, mistakenly, that true nutritive value can only come from whole foods, not nutritional supplements like protein powders and the like.

That is utter nonsense, which is not merely my opinion. Countless clinical studies have been performed on nutritional supplements (including protein powders) showing that they confer clear benefits beyond any reasonable doubt.

One recent study directly examined the effectiveness of protein supplementation versus whole food protein consumption.[8] In this study, researchers (Paul Arciero et. al.) divided chubby but otherwise healthy participants into two groups: One group that consumed six solid ("protein-paced") meals per day and another that consumed three solid protein-containing meals plus three protein shakes (in this case, from whey protein powder) per day.

Both groups consumed the same total number of calories, as well as the same total quantity of protein (1.4 grams per kilogram of body weight), and both performed the same workouts. After sixteen weeks, the researchers then analyzed changes in the participants' body composition.

The results of the study concluded that there were equal improvements in body composition between the two groups. It's my opinion that if a more specialized protein powder (blend) had been used, rather than just plain whey protein, the tie would have been broken in favor of the protein shake group.

Here's why:

- A blend of whey protein (preferably whey protein *isolate*) and micellar casein (*not* calcium or sodium caseinates, which are chemically-treated, inferior forms of casein) would have the distinct advantage of naturally possessing a timed-release quality in the way it supplies amino acids to muscle tissue (whey delivers amino acids relatively rapidly, while micellar casein delivers amino acids slowly for a period of up to seven hours, ensuring that both

protein synthesis is maximized and protein breakdown is
minimized)

- Due to its slow digestion rate and steady supply of amino
  acids, micellar casein is an overall better muscle builder
  than whey protein because of its scientifically-proven
  ability to maximize nitrogen retention (essential to muscle
  building) over other forms of protein, and it's natural
  anti-catabolic (muscle-sparing) effect[9]

While the nutritional supplement industry itself should be held
responsible for the view that nutritional supplements are
worthless (because so many companies don't invest in research or
quality products and rely instead on clever marketing hype to
sell them), the concept of supplementing your diet with quality,
convenient nutrition is a remarkably sound one, and should not
be discounted on the basis that many supplement companies are
unscrupulous.

For me, using protein powder and protein bars are utterly
essential because of their convenience, and moreover are
important "nice-haves" because I choose particular protein
supplements that outperform whole foods for both muscle
performance and muscle growth.

POST-WORKOUT NUTRITION

Aside from meal frequency, which we already covered, there is
another aspect to nutrient timing that I would be remiss not to
address: workout nutrition.

Of all the things that confound and frustrate gym goers from all
walks of life, it is probably this subject that takes the top

spot. Sometimes referred to as "peri-workout" nutrition (the prefix "peri" means "about" or "around"), the timing of nutrients before, during and after a workout has become something of an obsession among trainers, coaches and ordinary lifters, not to mention the supplement industry that spawned hundreds of workout nutrition products to capitalize on the frenzy.

So I'm going to cut through the confusion for you and set the record straight, once and for all.

First: forget about **pre-workout nutrition**, unless you're dragging ass on any given day and need something stimulatory to propel you through a workout. In that case, it wouldn't be inappropriate to consume a rational dose of caffeine or some other CNS stimulant about 30 minutes before starting your workout.

However, I recommend avoiding the consumption of protein or carb formulas during that time (pre-workout). Here's why:

- Some studies have concluded that consuming carbs within several minutes of a workout produces a rapid rise in blood glucose (sugar) and plasma insulin, resulting in a "sugar crash" when exercise begins. Obviously, this will hamper your performance.

- Consuming carbs too close to a workout interferes with normal glycogen and fat-mobilizing processes necessary to fuel your workout (caused by the insulin spike mentioned above). This will both lower performance and impair your body's ability to burn fat.

- Because exercise slows digestion and the absorption of nutrients, unabsorbed sugar in your stomach will not only be unavailable for use, but also produce negative osmotic effects on your body that, again, will hamper performance.

- Lest you think that only carbohydrates trigger the body to produce insulin (and thus produce the effects stated above), protein is also insulinotropic and can have the same effect if consumed too close to a workout.[10]

Recommendation: Ensure that there's at least 60 minutes between your last protein and carb feeding and when you start training.

Next: only supplement with certain nutrients during a workout in specific instances. Namely:

- Depending on the intensity and volume of your workout, glycogen (your body's stored form of energy [carbs]) can deplete rapidly. When it's substantially depleted, protein has to supply between 10% and 15% of the total energy demanded by your workout (up from just 5% when glycogen stores are normal), which means that muscle breakdown can start to occur. Therefore, ingesting simple carbs (like dextrose) *during* your workout to quickly replenish glycogen can be a great idea.

- Because your muscles have such a high demand for glycogen replacement during exercise, any simple sugars ingested at that time will be shuttled to muscles so quickly that the insulinogenic issues noted above (in the "pre-workout" section) do not occur.[10]

Recommendation: If you're so inclined, do feel free to supplement with dextrose (straight glucose) or an interesting "designer" carbohydrate like highly branched cyclic dextrin during a workout to replenish glycogen and reduce muscle protein breakdown. To take this to the next level, you can also combine

this carb drink with electrolytes to enhance uptake at the
muscle cell.

Lastly, and most importantly: DO follow a very precise post-
workout protocol consisting of the following (these figures are
for both men and women):

- Protein: ½ calorie per pound of bodyweight
- Carbohydrates: 1 calorie per pound of bodyweight
- Fats: 0 or as close to 0 as possible
- Creatine monohydrate: 5 grams

Yes, we're back to formulas again, but in the case of workout
nutrition, this level of precision is matched appropriately to
priority.[11] It's simply too important to treat willy nilly.

Within 30 minutes after your workout, I strongly recommend a
post-workout nutrition shake that contains a blend of:

1. **Whey protein** (preferably from whey protein isolate and/or
   hydrolyzed whey protein isolate -- not whey protein
   concentrate) to immediately kick start protein synthesis
   (muscle repair and rebuilding), and

2. **Micellar casein** (not sodium or calcium caseinates) to
   maximize leucine concentration and nitrogen retention over
   the subsequent 7-8 hours.

3. **Dextrose** (sometimes called D-glucose) to spike insulin,
   which in turn will replenish glycogen and transport vital
   nutrients to the muscle cell

4. **Creatine monohydrate** to maximize cell volume and trigger
   muscle anabolism

Using the formulas provided above, let's use our hypothetical 200-lb. male lifter again. His shake macros would look like this:

Protein: ½ calorie x 200 lbs. = 100 calories x .25 = **25 grams**
Carbohydrates: 1 calorie x 200 lbs. = 200 calories x .25 = **50 grams**
Fats: 0
Creatine: 5 grams

(Note that protein and carbohydrates consist of 4 calories per gram, which is why we need to multiply calories by .25 or 25% to convert them to grams.)

You'll also notice that the amount of protein is exactly half of the carbohydrate quantity, or another way to view it is that total carbs equals exactly 2 times the quantity of protein. This makes things simpler when planning your shake macros. Simply multiply your bodyweight by .25 to determine how much protein you need in grams, and then double that to determine the carb quantity in grams. Then simply add 5 grams of creatine, and you're ready to drink!

Easy, right?

Q: YOU SAID I DON'T HAVE TO COUNT CALORIES, SO WHY AM I CALCULATING ALL THESE NUMBERS?!

While counting calories is mostly futile in the long run, I do believe that you need to quantify calories and macronutrients when designing your nutrition plan. Then you can virtually "set it and forget it."

Because once you have determined what and (approximately) how much you are going to eat each day (on both maintenance and above-maintenance days), then the rest falls into place without your having to be concerned about weighing foods, counting calories and the like.

Obviously, you're going to want to vary your menu, and every time you make a tweak you'll want to re-consider calories and

macros, but thankfully, there is a really simple rule of thumb
that makes it easy:

A portion size of protein (P), carbohydrates (C) and fats (F)
would be approximately equal to:

    P = size of your clenched fist
    C = size of the palm of your hand
    F = size of your index finger

Thus, if your original menu was designed with 1 portion of
sirloin for dinner, but today you want to eat chicken breast,
then you would simply replace the beef with a piece of chicken
breast approximately equal in size to your clenched fit.

That's pretty easy, right?

Q: WHY IS IT RECOMMENDED THAT I ALTERNATE BETWEEN 100% AND 125% OF "MAINTENANCE" CALORIES?

Remember, your nutrition goal is to support maximum increases in
strength and lean body mass without gaining fat. To optimize
muscle growth without the use of powerful repartitioning agents
like anabolic steroids, you would need to consistently consume
more calories than your body burns in order to satisfy the
additional energy demand of the muscle-building process. The
problem with that, of course, is that constantly being in a
calorie-surplus state will lead to substantial body fat
accumulation over time because some of the excess calories with

neither be burned nor used to build muscle. The body's other
option is depositing excess calories into fat cells, its
evolutionary storage depot.

But, you can substantially skirt this problem by making a
compromise. Instead of elevated calorie intake *every* day,
alternating every other day between maintenance calories (the
quantity that theoretically maintains your body weight without
loss or gain) and 125% of maintenance calories will supply your
body with extra calories on a fairly regular basis without doing
so in perpetuity (which is ultimately the signal that instructs
the body to "switch priorities" over to fat storage).

In fact, a number of scientific studies have shown that "acute,"
or short-term overfeeding (consuming more calories than you
burn), leads initially to (substantial) lean body mass gains,
even among sedentary people who do not train with weights. This
favorable condition only lasts for about two weeks, however,
after which the body appears to abruptly change objectives and
begins to preferentially store fat.[12,13]

Thus, very modestly overfeeding on an every-other-day schedule
is a kind of dietary sleight-of-hand intended to optimize your
metabolism toward your goal of gaining attractive lean muscle
without sabotage from fat accumulation.

Q: I HAVE A HARD-ENOUGH TIME ON SOME DAYS JUST EATING 3 MEALS/DAY. HOW AM I GOING TO EAT 6?

I admit, six meals a day for some folks will be a challenge.
You might have an occupation that requires you to be on your

feet all day with limited time for breaks, or share office space
with people who are going to disapprove of the odor emanating
from your salmon and eggs.

But nobody said that building an extraordinary physique is going
to be easy, and a big part -- perhaps the biggest part -- of
excelling in anything is being willing to do what others are
not. If you're truly committed, you *will* find a way to get your
six meals in. It's simply a function of how resolute you are.

That said, here are my tips for making it easier:

- Don't buy into the "food purist" trend and uncritically
  swear off protein powders. The best trick for making six
  meals a day very closely resemble three meals a day is to
  use protein shakes for three of your six meals. That way,
  you're still only preparing/cooking/eating food for three
  meals, and simply chugging down a protein shake (which
  these days can taste like dessert if you're choosy) for the
  other three. Now, I've often heard the argument from folks
  that if only they had the budget for consuming 3 shakes a
  day, they certainly would, but that requires buying a lot
  of protein powder. To that I say, your alternative is
  doubling the size of your grocery bill. Which do you think
  is more expensive? Go ahead and break out the calculator
  if you don't believe me. You will *save* money by buying
  lots of protein powder, even if you opt for the good stuff
  over the discount powders found at all the big retail
  chains.

- Prepare your food in advance. I can't emphasize this
  enough. If you're going to stick to a consistent meal
  plan, especially one that includes six meals a day, it's
  difficult to get around having to prepare some of them in
  advance. Most people who work Monday through Friday find
  that preparing their weekly meals on Sunday works out very
  well for them, and it's not that hard or time consuming.

Cooking once in bulk and then packaging for the week is much more efficient than cooking dozens of times throughout the week on the fly.

- Eat nutrient- and calorie-dense foods. By this I mean, try to select foods that deliver all the goods without being really voluminous. For example, you can cover your carb requirement from a sweet potato and a handful of greens, or a giant cauldron of asparagus large enough to house a hibernating bear. If you tend toward having a large appetite, then focus primarily on nutrient density and opt for foods that take up a lot of space on your plate while delivering few calories. But if you're simply looking to meet your nutritional requirements with the least amount of food and effort, then the first option is the clear winner.

Q: DO I HAVE TO FOLLOW THE SAMPE MENUS AND EAT THE SAME FOODS?

No, of course not! I included two examples of my typical daily menu just to give you a practical, real-life illustration of what your nutrition plan can look like. Often, these concepts are abstract until you see them implemented. Now, if you're a male with similar body mass (roughly 200 lbs) and the sample menus reflect foods you would enjoy eating, then by all means go ahead and follow them precisely. Otherwise, feel at liberty to change it up and customize as much as you like to suit your particular preferences.

Q: HOW IMPORTANT IS THE POST-WORKOUT SHAKE YOU RECOMMEND?

While I don't consider the post-workout shake to be vital to your success (it's clearly not as important as, say, training hard and being consistent), I do believe it is hands-down the most important single "meal" of your day. This is because there is a rare, well-established window of opportunity following a weight training workout during which the consumption of protein and high-glycemic simple sugars kick starts a process of muscle tissue repair and rebuilding, which persists for a period of several hours. This is not conjecture, but established fact, which scientific study after study has confirmed beyond a reasonable doubt. If you properly take advantage of this opportunity with the right milieu of nutrients, you *will* build more muscle and get better results faster from your workouts, plain and simple. If you follow the guidelines I outlined above under "Workout Nutrition," you can rest assured that your workout nutrition strategy will be optimized for best results.

BONUS CHAPTER: 5-Star Supplements ★ ★ ★ ★ ★

I'm a big proponent of using nutritional supplements to improve performance, build muscle and recover more quickly from intense training.

Make no mistake, using nutritional supplements produces results that often pale in comparison to those experienced with performance-enhancing drugs, but with the right choices, they WILL make a difference in your training and physique. Used effectively, they can be an incredibly powerful tool for improving training outcomes.

I use and recommend the following:

- **High-quality protein powder**: It shouldn't be news to you that a high-protein diet is the foundation of a strength athlete's nutrition. It is generally suggested that weight training athletes should ingest a protein intake of up to 1 gram of protein per pound of body weight (and more in some instances).[14] For a 200-lb athlete, for example, this equates to at least 200 grams of protein.

Now, a word of caution concerning protein supplements: there are countless protein powders on the supplement market, and in my view, after immersing myself in the industry as a proprietor of a custom formulation, a very high percentage of commercially available proteins are mediocre or worse. Protein supplement quality, after peaking in the early- to mid-90's with a couple very innovative products that don't even exist today with the same high-quality formulas, has *generally* been on the decline for some time. During this time, there have been very substantial enhancements in protein technology and manufacturing methods that should have resulted in increasingly better products, but unfortunately the supplement companies decided to prioritize profit margins over quality and effectiveness, opting instead for mediocre protein sources and hyping them to the public as being much better than they are. It's a very effective formula, and one I ask you to be aware of when selecting a protein powder. Flashy graphics on labels and big, unsupported marketing claims don't equate to effective products, and are often warning signs that the products' results don't speak for themselves.

So, what should you look for?

In general, look for dairy protein isolates (whey and casein) produced with the industry's best extraction technologies, such as cross-flow micro- and nano-filtration. With respect to casein in particular, insist on micellar casein rather than the cheap (calcium or sodium) caseinates so often used in powders today.

(Note that one of casein's best features for strength athletes is that it promotes superior "nitrogen retention," a function of its characteristically slow digestion rate.[15] However, most casein supplements use sodium and calcium caseinates in their formulas, which result from chemically treating micellar casein (the natural form) to produce a wholesale-friendly low cost. The problem with that is that caseinates do not have slow digestion rates like undenatured casein.[17] Chemically altering the casein eradicates the "micelles" from which the digestion rate -- and nitrogen retention benefits -- arise, making the casein useless as a "timed-release" formula so often claimed by manufacturers of cheap casein. This is why you should never buy a casein supplement that doesn't derive all its casein from "micellar" casein.)

Also, I advise you NOT buy protein powders that contain formulas with a laundry list of inactive or questionable ingredients, free form amino acids (such as glutamine, taurine, etc.), and undisclosed "proprietary blends," as these are industry tricks for reducing potency and production costs, and ultimately selling you empty promises instead of high-quality complete proteins.

More basically, run everything through the sniff test. If the claims seem exaggerated, they usually are. Use your best judgment, and understand that as a rule, supplement companies are looking to make a buck first, and deliver value second (or not at all). This is NOT how business should be conducted, but unfortunately, it is the current state of the industry. It profits on consumer naïveté.

▪ **<u>Creatine</u>**: Second only to protein supplementation, creatine is another nutritional supplement that belongs in the arsenal of every strength (and endurance) athlete. Unlike many popular nutritional products today, creatine is backed by a plethora of concrete scientific research, which continues to conclusively demonstrate its ability to improve athletic performance and build muscle and strength. There's a growing body of evidence demonstrating its plentiful health benefits as well, ranging from improving brain power to reducing inflammation and even extending lifespan.[16] I use 5 grams of creatine on non-training days (in a single dose with my breakfast protein shake), and 10 grams on training days (divided into two doses, one with breakfast and the other with my post-workout shake).

▪ **<u>BCAAs ("branched chain amino acids")</u>:** Supplementing your diet with branched-chain amino acids (i.e leucine, isoleucine and valine) -- especially in the form of di- and tri-peptides, which are more effective at supporting increases in muscle than "free form" BCAAs) -- has well-documented benefits for strength athletes, including gains in strength, lean muscle and fat loss.[17,18,19] While many protein powders in today's market are "fortified" with free form aminos (that is, amino acids that are delivered individually rather than as part of complete proteins), I recommend that you absolutely do NOT supplement with BCAAs this way. The reason is beyond our scope, but I'll say that it gives supplement manufacturers a very enticing – and often irresistible – opportunity to reduce product costs and jack up profit margins by taking advantage of certain supplement label loopholes. To avoid this, I suggest using a high-quality BCAA supplement (preferably in capsule or tablet form, as the powder tastes absolutely offensive) as part of your workout nutrition strategy (i.e. before, during and/or after a workout).

- **Natural testosterone boosters**: Particularly for aging strength athletes (although any weight training male over 25 would certainly benefit), the importance of naturally supporting testosterone production speaks for itself. While there are a lot of purported test boosters on the supplement market, many are bunk; however, a handful are not, and can result in a significant increase in free testosterone levels ("free" testosterone, as opposed to "total" testosterone, is the active form responsible for testosterone's benefits). These are:

  o **DIM (Diindolylmethane)**: DIM is a metabolite of Indole-3-Carbinol (I3C), found in vegetables such as Brussels sprouts, broccoli, kale and others. It supports healthy testosterone production primarily through its actions on estrogen and the testosterone binding proteins.[20] At low doses, it also exhibits an inhibitory effect on the aromatase enzyme that converts testosterone to estrogen, resulting in higher levels of circulating free testosterone. Finally, its action on estrogen *per se* has direct benefits to strength athletes (such as by converting more potent forms to less potent forms). Doses of 200-300mg per day for males, and 100-200mg per day for females appear to maximize these effects.

- **ZMA (zinc, magnesium and vitamin B6):** Given relatively common zinc and magnesium deficiencies in the general population, and even more so among athletes, a number of scientific studies have demonstrated substantial performance gains by supplementing with a zinc, magnesium and vitamin B6 mineral-support formula. In fact, increases in free testosterone of 30% or more have been observed.[21] Additionally, ZMA is purported to significantly improve the quality of REM sleep, aiding workout recovery.

- **Fenugreek:** A popular herb native to Arabic regions, fenugreek is often used to enhance libido and increase testosterone, actions supported by several well-designed research studies.[22] Additionally, fenugreek also remarkably improves glucose metabolism, which is believed to explain the statistically significant reductions in body fat noted by researchers in the above-mentioned studies.

- **Tribulus terrestris:** Tribulus has been around for a while, which in this case is a testimonial to its efficacy for naturally increasing testosterone. It does this by increasing luteinizing hormone (LH), which is a hormone produced by the pituitary gland that stimulates the Leydig cells of the testes to produce testosterone. I typically use a 1,000mg daily dose concentrated to at least 20% saponins (i.e. 200mg of saponins, the active ingredients).

o **Tongkat ali (also called eurycoma longifolia)**: This is an interesting herb that is sometimes referred to as a pro-fertility agent and aphrodisiac, with anti-estrogen properties. It also appears to increase testosterone by converting dehydroepiandrosterone (DHEA), a precursor to testosterone, and other androgens to testosterone. Moreover, studies on young, healthy males showed tongkat ali produced greater gains in lean body mass (including arm circumference) from weight training.[23] I use 400mg daily of a 1:100 potency extract.

o **Maca root**: Also a purported fertility-enhancer and aphrodisiac, maca appears to lead to an increase in testosterone production by deactivating sex hormone binding globulin (SHBG), which otherwise binds to testosterone and renders it biologically inactive. I use 750mg daily of a 6:1 concentration.

o **Resveratrol**: This red wine derivative has been associated with the purported health benefits of red wine (including life extension). It also increases LH and follicle-stimulating hormone (FSH), which reduces the conversion of testosterone to estrogen via the aromatase enzyme as part of the feedback loop regulating testosterone production.[24] A reduction in this conversion equates to increased free testosterone levels. I use 250mg daily.

▪ **Fish oil**: The benefits of essential fatty acids (EFAs), particularly omega-3 fatty acids, are well documented. Like creatine, the benefits span the spectrum from overall health improvement to enhancements in athletic performance and body composition. I use fish oil daily for all of these reasons, but one, in particular, is vital to my ability to train at a high level week in and week out: fish oil is anti-inflammatory. Reducing inflammation after training is a key factor in recovery, and fish oil is a powerful anti-inflammatory agent, as useful as over-the-counter pain killers, without the side effects (one of which is the inhibition of protein synthesis, which can significantly thwart your muscle-building efforts!).[25] A couple grams of fish oil per day is sufficient to achieve these desired outcomes.

- **Forskolin**: This is a very interesting, and remarkably effective, nutritional supplement. It is produced via extraction from the roots of the coleus forskohlii plant. Although oral ingestion results in relatively poor absorption, using a concentrated supplement containing 25-50 mg doses of forskolin is sufficient to derive impressive health, physique and performance benefits.[26] Among these are the following:

  o **Body composition improvements**: Forskolin has been shown in research studies to produce fat loss (which is its most famous attribute), but also to increase lean body mass. This makes forskolin a great "cutting" supplement for natural bodybuilders.

  o **Increase testosterone production in males**: Forskolin increases the body's production of an enzyme called cyclic adenosine monophosphate (cAMP), which is associated with elevated fat-loss and testosterone production

- o **<u>Reduce blood pressure</u>**: I use forskolin primarily for its effectiveness in naturally reducing high blood pressure, which I inherited (thanks dad!). I use 50 mg a day for this purpose, and it reduces my blood pressure down to the high-end of "normal," without pharmaceuticals.

- o **<u>Other general health benefits</u>**: While these claims are more conjecture than those above, forskolin, nevertheless, has been noted as an effective treatment for allergies, various skin conditions (e.g. eczema, psoriasis, etc.), irritable bowel syndrome, urinary and bladder infections, and many others.

- **<u>Vitamin D3 (cholecalciferol)</u>**: Let me say that a diet rich in micronutrients, including, of course, vitamins and minerals, is vital to health and athletic performance. The reason I specifically break out vitamin D is because, for strength athletes, it's particularly powerful and, in my view, should be a core supplement. Here's why:

  - o **<u>Athletic performance enhancement</u>**: A metabolite of vitamin D (calcitrol) is a "secosteroid," which is a hormone similar in nature to a steroid. Vitamin D's production of this hormone is believed to be associated with its performance enhancing capabilities, which are well documented.

- o **Life extension**: A study published in the New England Journal of Medicine warned that a myriad of diseases are associated with vitamin D deficiency, and another study found that mortality rates were 26% higher in sample populations with the lowest vitamin D levels compared with the highest.

- o **Body composition**: It is believed that low levels of vitamin D may contribute to metabolic pathologies such as "syndrome X," diabetes and obesity.

I use 5000 IU of vitamin D3 per day.

- **Curcumin:** More than simply a sports nutrition supplement, curcumin should be regarded as a must-have health supplement. Its benefits have been recorded by scientists for decades, and it appears that curcumin positively affects every major organ system in your body. For strength athletes, however, it is especially interesting. Here are some of the highlights for serious lifters:

  - o Reduces post-workout delayed onset muscle soreness
  - o Is a potent anti-inflammatory without interfering with muscle growth (unlike many other anti-inflammatory agents)
  - o Increases insulin sensitivity and reduces body fat
  - o Helps prevent muscle loss during calorie-restrictive diets
  - o Increases testosterone levels in men (mild but measurable)
  - o Supports join health
  - o Improves gut health

I use approximately 1,000 mg a day of a 95% total
curcuminoid formula. Make sure it is combined with 5-10 mg
of piperine, which dramatically improves absorption.

Learn More

I urge you to always maintain an open mind, and continually
identify as a student before an expert. (The best experts are
lifelong students themselves.) There are many self-purported
experts citing an array of credentials to compete for your
attention, some of them sincere, many of them disingenuous and
motivated principally by profits. Either way, after more than
25 years of training and lots of self-discoveries, I will say
that ultimately you need to determine what works best for
yourself, and perhaps the best way to do this is by continuing
to learn from as many relevant sources as possible (look,
especially, outside the bubble), and especially from yourself.
Over time, you'll learn what works for YOU, as well as what
doesn't, and you'll be able to develop or modify strategies
accordingly.

Above all, don't allow the power of beliefs to eclipse your
ability to reason. Many accepted truths and staples of
conventional wisdom have been overturned throughout history
based on new evidence, insights and developments. Always keep
your mind open to new findings, and question dogma in all forms.

Lastly - be persistent! Beyond the next 12 weeks, I encourage
you to consider powerbuilding a life-long pursuit and a
lifestyle, not simply a periodic "shape-up" or strength program.

If you have any questions concerning training or nutrition, feel
free to reach out to me at **todd@powerbuildingblueprint.com**.

<u>Works Cited</u>

1. <u>Schoenfeld, Brad J. "The Mechanisms of Muscle Hypertrophy and Their Application to Resistance Training." Journal of Strength and Conditioning Research, vol. 24, no. 10, 2010, pp. 2857-2872., doi:10.1519/jsc.0b013e3181e840f3.</u>

2. <u>Zatsiorsky, Vladimir M., and William J. Kraemer. Science and Practice of Strength Training. Human Kinetics, 2006.</u>

3. <u>Hortobágyi Tibor, et al. "The Effects of Detraining on Power Athletes." Medicine & Science in Sports & Exercise, vol. 25, no. 8, 1993, doi:10.1249/00005768-199308000-00008.</u>

4. <u>Lammert, et al. Effects of isoenergetic overfeeding of either carbohydrate or fat in young men. Br J Nutr. 2000 Aug;84(2):233-45.</u>

5. <u>Genome Med. 2012 Nov 30;4(11):94. doi: 10.1186/gm395. eCollection 2012.</u>
<u>Assessing the metabolic effects of prednisolone in healthy volunteers using urine metabolic profiling. Ellero-Simatos S1</u>

6. <u>Am J Clin Nutr. 1996 Sep;64(3):259-66. Changes in macronutrient balance during over- and underfeeding assessed by 12-d continuous whole-body calorimetry. Jebb SA1, Prentice AM, Goldberg GR, Murgatroyd PR, Black AE, Coward WA.</u>

7. Am J Clin Nutr. 1989 Apr;49(4):608-11. Hormonal response to overfeeding. Forbes GB1, Brown MR, Welle SL, Underwood LE.

8. Nutrients. Paul J. Arciero, et al. Protein-Pacing from Food or Supplementation Improves Physical Performance in Overweight Men and Women: The PRISE 2 Study, May 2016.

9. J Sports Sci Med. 2004 Sep; 3(3): 118-130. International Society of Sports Nutrition Symposium, June 18-19, 2005, Las Vegas NV, USA - Symposium - Macronutrient Utilization During Exercise: Implications For Performance And Supplementation Protein - Which is Best? Jay R. Hoffman✉* and Michael J. Falvo*

10. Maria C. Linder (ed), Nutritional Biochemistry and Metabolism (Elsevier Press, New York, 1991).

11. Michael Colgan, Optimum Sports Nutrition (Advanced Research Press, New York, 1993)

12. Am J Clin Nutr. 1996 Sep;64(3):259-66. Changes in macronutrient balance during over- and underfeeding assessed by 12-d continuous whole-body calorimetry. Jebb SA1, Prentice AM, Goldberg GR, Murgatroyd PR, Black AE, Coward WA.

13. Am J Clin Nutr. 1989 Apr;49(4):608-11. Hormonal response to overfeeding. Forbes GB1, Brown MR, Welle SL, Underwood LE.

14.   Phillips, Stuart M., and Luc J.c. Van Loon. "Dietary Protein for Athletes: From Requirements to Optimum Adaptation." Journal of Sports Sciences, vol. 29, no. sup1, 2011, doi:10.1080/02640414.2011.619204.

15.   Boirie, Y., et al. "Slow and Fast Dietary Proteins Differently Modulate Postprandial Protein Accretion." Proceedings of the National Academy of Sciences, vol. 94, no. 26, 1997, pp. 14930-14935., doi:10.1073/pnas.94.26.14930; Wang, Xin, et al. "Gastric Digestion of Milk Protein Ingredients: Study Using an in Vitro Dynamic Model." Journal of Dairy Science, vol. 101, no. 8, 2018, pp. 6842-6852., doi:10.3168/jds.2017-14284.

16.   Cooper, Robert, et al. "Creatine Supplementation with Specific View to Exercise/Sports Performance: an Update." Journal of the International Society of Sports Nutrition, vol. 9, no. 1, 2012, doi:10.1186/1550-2783-9-33.

17.   Blomstrand E, Saltin B. – BCAA intake affects protein metabolism in muscle after but not during exercise in humans. Am J Physiol Endocrinol Metab. 2001 Aug;281(2):E365-74.

18.   Candeloro N, Bertini I, Melchiorro G, DeLorenzo A. – Effects of prolonged administration of branched chain amino acids on body composition and physical fitness. Minerva Endocrinol 1995;20(4):217-223.

19.   Mourier A, Bigard AX, deKerviler E, et al. - Combined effects of caloric restriction and branched chain amino acid supplementation on body composition and selected performance parameters in elite wrestlers. Int J Sports Med. 1997;18:47-55.

20.   Michael Zeligs, M.D. and A. Scott Connelly, M.D. All About DIM (Michael A. Zeligs, 2000 and 2008)

21.   Brilla, L. Effects of zinc-magnesium (ZMA) supplementation on muscle attributes of football players. ACSM journal, Medicine and Science in Sports and Exercise, Vol.31, No. 5, May 1999.

22.   Poole, Chris et al. "The effects of a commercially available botanical supplement on strength, body composition, power output, and hormonal profiles in resistance-trained males." *Journal of the International Society of Sports Nutrition* vol. 7 34. 27 Oct. 2010, doi:10.1186/1550-2783-7-34

23.   Hamzah S, Yusof A. The ergogenic effects of Tongkat ali (Eurycoma longifolia): A pilot study. British J Sports Med. 2003;37:464-470.

24.   Balunas, Marcy J et al. "Natural products as aromatase inhibitors." *Anti-cancer agents in medicinal chemistry* vol. 8,6 (2008): 646-82.

25.	Maroon, JC et al. "Omega-3 fatty acids (fish oil) as an anti-inflammatory: an alternative to nonsteroidal anti-inflammatory drugs for discogenic pain." *Surgical Neurology, Apr 2006 65(4);326-31.*

26.	Godard, Michael & A Johnson, Brad & Richmond, Scott. (2005). Body Composition and Hormonal Adaptations Associated with Forskolin Consumption in Overweight and Obese Men. Obesity research. 13. 1335-43. 10.1038/oby.2005.162.